Chicken Raising And Caring

Raising Backyard Chickens for Beginners

Norman Nelson

PUBLISHED BY:
Norman Nelson
Copyright © 2012

Preparing the Chicken Coop for Winter

Chapter 4   : Tips on how to sanitize your chicken coop

Sanitizing the Chicken Coop

How Do You Clean the Chicken Coop

What products are good to use to clean the coop?

How can you get rid of flies from pestering your chicken coop?

How do you keep the dust to a minimum inside the coop?

How many times do you need to clean your coop in a day? Or week?

Chapter 5   : Tips in Choosing the Right Breed for Egg Production or for Chicken Meat

Criteria for Choosing the Best Breed of Chicken for Egg Production

Number of eggs

Color of eggs

Best egg layers

Breeds that are both good egg layers and good for meat

Smaller breeds

Criteria in choosing the breed best for chicken meat produce?

Chicken breeds for flavor

Easiest and most useful breed for producing meat

Free Range Chickens

Most popular breed for poultry producers

What type of breed is hardy and appropriate for the Northeast winter/summer extreme climate?

Breeds for cold weather

Breeds for hot weather

Introduction

This eBook is a comprehensive guide to raising chickens. You will learn all you need to know about how to manage a back yard flock. Every chicken has a personality and they are quite sociable birds. They make surprisingly good pets but are also very useful as a low cost supply of meat and eggs.

This guide will tell you the best breeds for eggs and meat. Plus you will be able to get the best breeds for your area that can survive the extremes of severe winters.

Chickens are not only good for eggs and meat but will help you with your yard. Their droppings make great fertilizer and when they forage they will aerate your garden and get rid of pests in the yard. They can be put in a tractor coop and wheeled to any part of your garden that needs clearing and preparation for planting.

There are low cost ways to make your own feed and methods to ensure that you can raise them organically without the aid of commercial feeds. You will find recipes for chick feed and chicken feeds that will allow you to make sure your meat and eggs are organic and your chickens will be happy and healthy.

Raising chickens is not as hard as people think and is very rewarding. You will get eggs that are more nutritious and better tasting than any store bought eggs. Plus you can have the luxury of having organic meat and eggs without the high cost of organic food.

Cleanliness is the key to success and you will learn how to look after your birds without spending a lot of time. You will find helpful tips and methods for keeping your chicken coop clean. This is something that many people think is hard to do as chickens are considered a rather dirty animal but it is much easier than you think. There are tips and techniques in this guide that you may not even have thought about.

Another area of concern is keeping the chickens laying well. There are lots of information for you to increase the quality and production of your eggs. Chickens are quite tough birds but there are some diseases that they can get. You will learn important information on how to care for them when they get sick and when to call the vet. It is surprising that many diseases that afflict chickens can be taken care of at home and many of them can be prevented by a little hygiene.

This is a guide that you will want to keep with you. It will inspire you to have fun and enjoy keeping back yard chickens.

Chapter 1: Know your chickens – behavior, breed and biology

Egg laying

This is one of the main reasons that people keep chickens. A home grown egg from free range chickens is one of the greatest rewards of raising chickens.

At what age do the chickens start laying eggs?

Chickens will start laying at around 6 months and some of the heavier breeds will take a little longer. The lighter breeds like leghorns and Australorps might start a little sooner

How long does an egg grow inside the hen before she lays it?

For many breeds it will take around 24 hours to develop an egg. Most breeds will lay one egg per day and other breeds will lay every three days.

How long do you have to wait before the eggs hatch?

It usually takes around 21 days for a chicken to hatch an egg. You should not allow a chicken to sit on more than 6 to 12 eggs at a time or they will have difficulty looking after them.

Do hens brood eggs only in a certain season or do they brood eggs all year round?

This will depend on the breed of chicken. Some breeds will brood a lot and others rarely. Officially the brooding season is March to September, when the weather is warmer. Silkies are good brooding hens and will sit on almost anything. Game birds are also good brooders and very good mothers. However, they are aggressive birds and need to be introduced to the flock when they are chicks.

Why do chickens have fewer eggs during the winter?

This has something to do with the chicken's metabolic make up. As the days get shorter, the egg production of the chicken will reduce. Colder weather will also effect the chicken's egg production. The way to keep up egg laying is to have a light in the coop where they lay their eggs. This tricks the chicken into thinking that the days are not getting shorter and she should continue to lay eggs. The coop should also be kept warm in winter.

For how many years do a chicken lay eggs?

This will depend on the breed. Poultry farms kill the chickens at around 2 years as they consider that the chicken's egg production will decrease after that time. However, a laying breed of hen will continue to lay eggs on a regular basis for up to 5 to 7 years. As hens begin to age they will lay fewer eggs.

How many eggs does a chicken lay in a day?

A chicken will lay around one egg a day and no more. Some breeds will lay every 3 days. Majority of hens will get their laying done before 10 am in the morning.

How long do chickens live?

Many people wonder how long a chicken will actually live if they are not slaughtered early by the factory farms.

Free range birds can live for 10 years and some have even been known to survive for 20 years. Of course they will lay fewer eggs after the age of two years. Meat hens will be slaughtered at 6 weeks. Factory farms will kill egg laying birds at 2 years when their egg laying capacity goes down.

Mating

For those who wish to breed their chickens here are some facts about chickens mating habits:

How do chickens mate?

The rooster hops on the back of the hen and holds the feathers of her neck with his beak. He then tucks his tail under the hen's tail and shoots his sperm into her cloaca. Roosters do not have external penises because everything is inside. They will decide how much sperm will be ejected into the hen. The sperm will last about 7 days. The Rooster will decide which hens are the best to mate with based on their overall health.

Do you need a rooster for the chickens to lay eggs?

You do not need a rooster for a hen to lay eggs. The hen will carry on laying eggs regardless of whether a rooster has fertilized them. However in order to have chicks, the eggs must be fertilized by the rooster.

How do you know a fertilized egg from an unfertilized one?

To tell whether an egg is fertile or not you can check by candling it. You simply hold the egg up to a candle and check whether it is fertile. The fertile egg will appear opaque and the infertile egg will be clear. There are special lights made for this purpose which you can also use.

Raising Chickens

Is it hard to raise chickens?

It is not that hard if you know a little about raising chickens and chose the right breed for your area.

The hardest part of raising chicken is taking care of the small chicks. They will need to be kept warm until they start to get their real feathers. For this you will need a heat lamp which can be purchased at your local feed store. You will also need to keep them clean on a daily basis. The next thing to consider is housing the chickens and protecting them from predators. You will also have to be sure that the chicken coop is kept warm in winter if you have severe winters. You then have to decide whether you will keep egg layers or meat chickens. A small flock of around 6 birds is good to start with. Some people with less space like to keep bantams. You can keep egg layers and meat birds together but should not cross breed them.

Can chickens, fowls and geese live together in a single coop?

Yes all these birds can live together. However, they need a good sized run to get exercise and freedom. If they remain cooped up without leaving the coop, they can have issues, especially guinea fowl.

At what age do chickens molt?

Sometimes when new chicken owners see the birds in molt they think something must be wrong. However this is a normal cycle for a chicken and there is no cause for alarm.

Chicks will molt at 1 to 6 weeks. They will have a partial molt at 12 to 16 weeks, 7 to 9 weeks and a final molt at 20 to 22 weeks. They will have their full feathers at this time. After the bird becomes mature at around 6 months, they will molt once a year.

Do roosters need to be separated from one another when they are with the pullets?

When roosters are chicks they get on just fine and will continue to be happy if they have grown up together. They will not have to be separated. However they will separate themselves into the dominant and subdominant roosters.

Chapter 2 : Advantages of Raising Your Own Chickens

History of Chicken Raising

Where did the domesticated chickens come from?

They came from a breed of bird known as the jungle red fowl. It is a breed of chicken and still exists today in the jungles of South East Asia. However, the characteristics of domestic chickens have changed. They are less aggressive, do not forage for food as much and are not as socially active. The domestic chicken has less fancy plumage and is a heavier bird. The eggs of the domestic bird are larger and they lay earlier and more frequently.

Who were the first people to keep domestic chickens?

The Chinese were the first known people to raise chickens. By 2,000 BC, the birds were raised in the Indus valley. They were then discovered by the Europeans and Africans. Archaeological sites in the New Kingdom of Egypt showed evidences of the first chicken raising in East Africa. The ancient Greeks did not raise chickens much but chicken raising became well-established in the Roman Empire. By 1500 AD chickens appeared in West Africa.

In the Americas, chickens were first raised by settlers in Chile in 1350. This evidence contradicts the popular theory that these birds were brought to the Americas by the Spanish conquistadors. The birds that were raised here are a breed called the Araucana. This bird has little tufts of feathers on the face termed as ear tufts. It lays bluish colored eggs and the modern breed can also lay pinkish colored eggs. This is because the original Araucana chicken was crossbred with the Quetro. This bird does not have facial tufts and lays pinkish eggs. The modern day Araucana resembles the Americana breed.

The advantages of raising your own chickens

- Healthier eggs: There is no doubt about the fact that the eggs gathered from your own backyard flock are more nutritious and better for you. This is because commercial feed for chickens is of minimal nutrition and is merely given to the chicken to help her lay eggs.

Free range chickens raised by you have better feed and you can ensure that they receive a good nutritious diet.

- The eggs will taste better: You can definitely tell the difference from a store bought egg and a free range one from your own yard. It will taste better. The yolks of home raised chickens are dark yellow, indicating the presence of more iron and nutrition.

- You will save more: You can have the advantage of organic eggs and meat when you raise the chickens at home without having to pay exorbitant prices.
- The eggs are fresh: In the store the eggs may say they are fresh but could have waited several days before they get to the grocery store. Eggs from your own back yard can be gathered and eaten the same day.

- The chicken droppings will enrich your compost and produce very good fertilizer for your garden. This will help you to grow great organic fruits and vegetables.

- When they scratch around for tasty morsels they will scratch up the soil and aerate it. The soil will be a great consistency for your plants.

- They will eat pests and keep these annoying insects out of the garden. Chickens will eat a great deal of insects in your garden and will drop their stool while foraging.

- Chickens are entertaining. If ever you had the time to observe your chickens, you will see that each one has a special character and there is a certain hierarchy among them called the pecking order.

- They are good learning tools for children. It is good for children to learn how to look after chickens and know that eggs were not grown in the store. Looking after animals will increase a child's sense of responsibility.

How many chickens do you need to start with when you want to have your own poultry?

This will depend on your egg consumption. You should start with at least 2 birds as hens are quite sociable. Remember that most egg laying breeds will lay around 1 egg a day so you will be able to calculate the egg production based on this. The chickens will lay for about nine months then stop laying in the winter months. To get around 7 eggs per day you will need around 8 to 12 chickens.

As the birds get older, they will lay bigger eggs but they will not be as many as when they were young. If you want to keep the eggs laying production on a regular basis, you should get some new pullets every spring. Alternatively, you can keep some brooders like Silkies and keep some pullets back from the clutch to replenish your stock and keep egg production at a maximum.

If you are keeping the chickens for meat then you should consider how much meat you want and keep as many meat chickens as you will need. You can replenish these from your breeding stock. It is good to keep meat birds for breeding away from those that are being breed for eggs.

Chapter 3 : Efficient Ways to Keep the Temperature of the Coop Right for the Chickens

Keeping the Chickens Warm for the Winter

Do you need a heat or light bulb in your chicken house during the winter?

This will all depend on your climate. If you have mild winters where the temperatures do not plunge below freezing then you will not have to have any heat in the coop. However, you may still want to give some light to the chicken house to keep up egg production. The hens will need at least 14 hours of light to continue laying. You can use any light for this purpose.

If your winters are severe it is good to have a heat light in the coop. Chickens are not very smart and can burn themselves with the light or peck at it and cause it to break. Therefore the light needs to be away from them and hung on the roof about six feet high. You can place a wire cage of chicken wire around the bulb to prevent any accidents. One lamp to 6 to 10 chickens is a good ratio and will keep the coop warm.

How warm should the chicken coop be in the winter?

The coop should be kept at 50 degrees to 60 degrees in winter. The birds will often produce quite a bit of heat as they fluff themselves out at night when they roost.

How do you keep your chickens warm during the winters?

A light can keep them warm as mentioned above.

Chickens fluff out their feathers and produce quite a bit of heat when they roost. So they will produce warmth in the coop in winter. They also like to roost at night and will huddle close to each other to keep each other warm. They will need at least 4 square feet of space per bird and roosts should be around 2 feet off the ground.

Deep litter will keep the chickens warm. You can keep the coop heated by starting with a clean coop and laying down 4 inches of litter in the beginning of the fall as the weather starts to get cooler. Add more bedding so that it will stay dry and clean. By the time the winter starts, the litter will be around 8 to 10 inches deep. As it rots down the warmth of the decomposing litter will produce warmth for the chickens. You should always have a little ventilation for the coop as humidity can get quite high with this method.

A feed of corn before the chickens turn in for the night will help to keep them warm. You can stop the chickens' water from freezing by buying a small heater that goes under their water container.

Can you heat a chicken coop with an underground heating system?

Yes this can be done and is a very efficient way to warm a chicken coop.

Here is how it works:

It uses heat that naturally occurs from the earth to heat an area. The heat is produced from the radioactive breakdown of matter. A small amount is generated from the earth's core and is conducted to the surface of the earth. The surface of the earth is naturally warmed by the atmosphere and sunshine. At 10 feet the earth maintains a temperature of around 50 degrees F or 10 degrees C. Heat pumps are used to extract the heat from the ground to warm the area. Pipes are placed beneath the coop floor to keep the coop warm. You will find that pipes closest to the surface will produce more heat from the ground.

Preparing the Chicken Coop for Winter

Your first task will be to clean everything in the coop. This will include nesting boxes and any shelving you may have to support the roosts. All feeding utensils should also be taken out and cleaned. You should also give the walls and floor a good cleaning. This will make sure you have a clean coop and get rid of any small predators and parasites.

Check all the old bedding for parasites and also check the birds. The birds should be checked on a regular basis and treated if they have any external parasites. Small creatures can also hide in the bedding and when you do your detailed cleaning you can flush these small animals out as well.

Put clean bedding down and remove all old damp bedding. This is very important if you are going to rely on deep litter to warm the coop in winter time. Put down 4 inches of fresh bedding. This can be hay or a mixture of wood shavings. Be sure you rake the bedding to be sure it is well-aerated.

Inspect the coop to be sure that it is weatherproof especially the roof. Be sure it is properly insulated but will still provide ventilation for the chickens. Ensure the coop is predator safe and there are no cracks and holes that the predators can enter through.

Chapter 4 : Tips on how to sanitize your chicken coop

Sanitizing the Chicken Coop

The key to good sanitization and making the coop smell better is keeping it clean. You should give the chicken's clean bedding at least once or twice per week. They should have fresh water and food every day. Try to make sure they are not crowded; a chicken needs space and should have around 8 feet per medium size bird.

Make sure that the coop is not leaking and especially check the roof. If there are any leaks the coop will get damp and smell. It is also not good for the health of your chickens.

Make sure that the coop is properly ventilated. If necessary make more holes and cover them with chicken wire to allow the air to pass through and ventilate the chicken pen. This will cut down humidity

How Do You Clean the Chicken Coop

Try to use natural products to clean the coop as this will not harm the chickens. Chemicals can produce eye and respiratory diseases which chickens are very susceptible to. A detailed weekly cleaning or light daily cleaning will keep the coop in good condition.

For a detailed cleaning you should rake out all the old bedding and clean the roosts. You can use a 50/50 solution of vinegar and water to sanitize the shelving and roosts. Once this has been done, you will be able to put clean dry bedding down. 4 inches of wood shavings or straw will be good for the chickens' bedding. You can use the old spoiled bedding for compost.

Clean the walls and floor with the vinegar solution. Scrub them well to get rid of dirt and poop. Do not forget the nesting boxes and roosts.

When you clean be sure to check the roosts and nesting boxes for mites and splinters, evidence of mites are blood spots and black marks. Put down a mix of herbs like lemon balm, mint, thyme, basil, bee balm, marigold, oregano, lavender, and rose petals. These herbs will act as anti bacterial, anti viral and also natural insecticides. They are also good for the health and well-being of the chickens. The herbs will also help to repel parasites and rodents from the coop.

What products are good to use to clean the coop?

Natural products are best for cleaning a coop. Chickens are surprisingly sensitive to chemicals and can easily get respiratory and eye problems. To keep your flock healthy, you can try to use some natural homemade recipes. As mentioned a 50/50 solution of vinegar and water is a good cleaner and disinfectant. You can also use some herbal recipes.

A rose scented cleaner can be used by mixing ¼ cup of rose petals, 1 tablespoon of salt and 1 cup of baking soda. Mix in blender and sprinkle on surface to be cleaned. You can use a little water and scrub the walls, floor and accessories of the coop.

This recipe is an all purpose cleaner that can be used on walls and floors etc: 6 cups of water, 1 cup liquid castile soap, ¼ cup of thyme leaf tea, ¼ cup lemon juice. The lemon juice is a good anti bacterial substance.

How can you get rid of flies from pestering your chicken coop?

Hanging bags of water with a penny in the bottom is said to repel flies. This is how it works. Flies have multiple eyes and the reflection of light on the water really confuses them and makes them go away.

Basil plants can also repel these pests. Grow a couple in pots and put them by the door of your coop and be sure they are protected from your chickens as they will eat them. Chickens will eat almost anything, so put some chicken netting around the plants to make them chicken proof. Flies do not like the smell of the strong basil and will keep away. Be sure to pinch them back when they are about 6 inches high, to ensure they do not flower.

Lemons are also good at repelling flies. You just cut one into quarters and steep in a pint of boiling water overnight. Put the liquid into a spray bottle and spray on the walls. It will keep the flies away and make the coop smell good.

How do you keep the dust to a minimum inside the coop?

To keep dust to a minimum inside the chicken coop you can clean out the coop every day, instead of once a week. Chickens are birds and are naturally dusty. However if you keep them clean and have a nice run for them, you can keep dust to a minimum. Do not use Diatomaceous Earth as it creates more dust. Keep bedding fresh and clean by removing and replacing with dry bedding once a week.

How many times do you need to clean your coop in a day? Or week?

Once a day is adequate if you want a super clean coop, otherwise you can clean everything in detail once a week. You can keep shelves underneath the roosts and take them out and clean them every day.

Chapter 5 : Tips in Choosing the Right Breed for Egg Production or for Chicken Meat

Criteria for Choosing the Best Breed of Chicken for Egg Production

Almost all small poultry farmers and just about everybody who raises chickens in their backyard are interested in having chickens that lay eggs. However, not all breeds of chickens are known for being good egg layers. Any female chicken can lay eggs that have the same nutritional value as any other but some are known for consistently laying eggs with superior qualities. No matter whether you have chickens for your own egg production or for commercial purposes it is important to consider a variety of factors in choosing your egg laying breed of chickens.

Number of eggs

If you are raising chickens for your own use, you may not want chickens that are the best at egg laying as they may actually produce more eggs than you can use. Top breeds for egg laying can lay up to 300 eggs per year.

Color of eggs

The color of eggs has become a topic of interest for consumers. In different sections of the United States such as the Northeast, brown shelled eggs are far more popular than the traditional white egg popular in the rest of the country. If you are into more colorful variations of eggs, there is a breed of chicken referred to as an Easter Egger though the American Poultry Association calls this breed the Ameraucana. Eggs produced by the Easter Egger or Easter Egg Chicken are shades of green to blue to pink. Some egg producers like to have a variety of chicken breeds that produce different colored eggs which are a novelty and popular in market outlets such as Farmers Markets. The American Poultry Association provides a list of each breed and the color of the egg they produce from brown to buff white, light brown, white, dark brown and rich brown.

Best egg layers

Breeds known for being good egg laying chickens include a variety of breeds but the Leghorn breed is considered to be the best of all breeds. In the United States, the eggs most often seen in grocery stores are from the Single Comb White Leghorn breed. These are the white eggs that you will see in the stores. Other good egg laying breeds include the Rhode Island Reds, the Red Star, the Light Sussex, the Black Star, the Plymouth Rock, the Red Star, the Barred Rock and the Cuckoo Maran. Rhode Island Reds and Barred Rocks will lay brown eggs.

Breeds that are both good egg layers and good for meat

If you are interested in producing both eggs for sale or home use in addition to raising chicken for meat, you may be interested in what is known as dual purpose chicken breeds. These are breeds of chicken that are good egg layers and the male chickens are good for meat. Breeds of chicken in this category include the Plymouth Rock, Wyandottes, and the Sussex.

Smaller breeds

Backyard farmers or larger commercial outfits may also want to consider bantam breeds. Almost all breeds of chickens come in both a standard size and a smaller size known as bantams. They are usually easier to handle and take less feed and require less physical space. In terms of eggs, the eggs are smaller but some consumers seem to prefer the smaller egg size.

Criteria in choosing the breed best for chicken meat produce?

Finding the right breed of chicken to start with if you are going to be raising chickens for meat can be difficult with all the breeds to choose from. Raising chickens is great way to begin producing your own meat for yourself or for sale. They take relatively little space and can be raised in a backyard or on a large farm.

Deciding on the best breed of chicken for your needs depends on a variety of things including your locale, whether you are only raising them for meat or is egg production also important. Once you have chosen your breed there are mail order hatcheries or you can look online to identify poultry breeders in your area.

There are several things to consider when choosing a breed of chicken for its meat quality. Items to consider include looking at the flavor of the meat, the growth rate for the breed, the mature size of the chicken, and feed efficiency. A recent survey which asked poultry breeders these types of questions determined that certain breeds were better in terms of flavor but they may not be the same breed that rates the highest in terms of size, feed efficiency and rate of growth. You will have to determine the most important factor to you in terms of breeds.

Chicken breeds for flavor

Breeds that ranked the highest for flavor as opposed to chicken you would find on a supermarket shelf included Buckeyes, Cornish, Dorkings and La Fleche which was ranked the highest.

Easiest and most useful breed for producing meat

Ranked in terms of a combination of size, rate of growth and the ability to convert feed on an efficient basis included Orpingtons, Plymouth Rocks, Cornish, Rhode Island Whites, and Buckeyes. The breeds that came out the best in all categories including flavor were the Buckeyes and the Cornish breeds.

Free Range Chickens

If you will be raising your chickens as free range chickens which means allowing them to graze on pasture then the best rated chickens who do well in a free range environment are the Minorca, Malay, Hamburg, Polish, Old English Game and Catalana breeds.

Most popular breed for poultry producers

The most popular breed that is raised for poultry meat by both commercial poultry companies and smaller farms is the Cornish White Rock cross breed. Most of the broilers found in supermarkets are this breed. The advantage of this breed for meat production is that there is an efficient feed conversion ratio. They grow fast, broad breasted or meatiness, and they have fewer feathers which make them easier to pluck. Grown in confinement as opposed to free range production, this breed of chicken will grow to a weight of five pounds in approximately seven weeks making them market ready. Their rapid growth can also mean a major increase in health problems in the breed including heart problems, low heat tolerance and frail legs which makes them less viable for use as free range or pasture produced chicken. Also because of their rapid growth if allowed to grow larger before being brought to market their health problems and weak legs are exacerbated. Poultry producers interested in pasture and free range chicken production are currently looking at different breeds that are better equipped to handle pasture production but still meet the standards for taste, and feed efficiency.

What type of breed is hardy and appropriate for the Northeast winter/summer extreme climate?

Raising chickens is a fun and worthwhile occupation or hobby but in order for your poultry enterprise to be successful, you have to pick the right breed for your locale. In addition to considering healthy egg production and feed efficiency, you also have to consider weather tolerance. When you get your chicks in the warm springtime, you may not be thinking about how they are going to tolerate the cold temperatures of winter or the hot humid summer. If you live in the Northeast United States, you are going to want to pick a hardy breed of chicken that tolerates the extremes of temperatures that occur in your region.

Breeds for cold weather

Breeds of chicken that are known to do well in cold weather include a variety of breeds including the Chanteclers, the Brahmas, the Javas breed and the Buckeyes. In general chicken breeds that possess small combs and wattles are more likely to do better in colder climates. The Chantecler is a breed that was developed to withstand the cold in Canada with its pea comb. Also the Buckeye breed was developed in Ohio where it does well.

Breeds for hot weather

For birds that will do the best in hot sultry weather, the chosen breeds are the Malays, Sumatras, Javas, the Cubalayas, and the Jungle Fowl. In warm climates that are both humid and high in temperatures, chickens that possess large wattles and combs which help dispel the heat do better. Note that the Javas breed of chicken is the only ones that are recommended for both extremes of cold and hot weather.

Birds making a comeback

The official state bird of Rhode Island, the Rhode Island Reds at one point were very popular as a breed of chickens. This breed is one to consider as it does very well in the cold and tolerates the heat. This breed is currently making a comeback particularly with the small chicken farmer. The Rhode Island Reds are considered to be good layers and their meat is also prized. Another bird that is growing in popularity which does well in New England weather is the New Hampshire Red. This dual purpose breed is known for its flavorful meat though it is not as good a layer as other birds.

The chicken coop

No matter which breed you pick to raise, if you live in the Northeast you will need to provide a chicken coop that will protect your poultry flock from the extreme weather. In addition to being as predator proof as you can make it, the coop needs to be strong and weather resistant. Your flock will depend on this coop to stay alive or they could die from exposure. The coop should provide shade during the hot summer months and shield the flock from rain. In the winter it needs to be draft proof and will require additional insulation.

Talk to your local chicken breeders to find out which breed of chicken does particularly well in your locale. There are local poultry breeders associations and clubs all around the Northeast area.

Chapter 6: Ways to Keep Pests/Predators away from Your Chickens

The natural predators of chickens

Most commercial poultry producers do not have a problem with predators getting to their chickens as most commercially raised chicken live in secure buildings made of concrete and a roof and any outside areas are totally enclosed. It is the small poultry farms with free range chickens and people who raise chickens in their backyards that have the most problem with losing their poultry to predators.

If you are raising chickens without an enclosed structure, it is pretty much a sure thing you will lose some of your chickens to predators.

Organic farmers who raise free range chickens that graze are at risk from predators. The economic losses for a small poultry farmer from predation can be severe. Providing chickens housing in buildings such as barns or sheds may not be sufficient to keep predators away. The most dangerous time for the chickens is at dusk and at night as this is the most common time for predators to hunt. The chickens do not see well at night and are easy prey for predators.

Which animals are the predators?

To be properly prepared to care for your poultry flock and keep them from predators, it is important to know the most common predators for your area. The type of animals depends on your specific locale as to what animal might show up to attack the chickens. Predators of poultry can include coyotes, raccoons, weasels, rats, skunks, snakes, bobcats, mountain lions, foxes, opossums, hawks, and owls. Minxes that have escaped from minx farms are also a predator. Domestic and feral cats can be a problem as well as domestic dogs.

Each type of predator has characteristic behaviors that you will need to protect the chickens from. It is in daytime when you have to worry about hawks and other birds of prey taking chickens. Hawks generally will go after small or young birds but have been known to disappear with an entire chicken. Putting a roof on the run can help with this problem.

Determining which predator is the problem

Once a predator has attacked your poultry flock it can be possible to determine the type of predator based on the type of attack. If it is a dog, they will not eat the chicken but just leave the carcass. If you find chickens missing their heads or limbs, it was probably an attack by raccoons that stretch through chicken wire to grab the chickens head. Minxes also decapitate the chicken in order to feast off their blood.

If you find chickens smothered to death it could any number of predators. If chickens panicked they can pile into a corner of a pen or enclosure and die from being smothered. If you are missing chicks or eggs it could be hawks, snakes, cats, rodents, opossums, or skunks. If you find wounded birds, take a look around for animals from the weasel family who tend to bite their prey.

Both domestic cats or dogs or feral cats can also be a problem for your poultry flock. Cats will attack chickens during the nighttime. Dogs should be considered a danger unless they have been around chickens for a long time without showing aggression. Of course, some dogs can be trained to protect your flock and other animals, an example of a natural predator becoming a protector.

How do you keep pest/predators away from your chickens?

Raising chickens for commercial purposes or hobby means you have to be ready to protect the chicken run and the chicken coop from every direction as there are natural predators just waiting to make off with a chick, egg or full grown chicken.

Large commercial producers of chickens don't usually have a problem with predators getting to their chickens due to the fact that most of them keep their poultry flock in secure buildings. An organic poultry farmer who wants his chickens to graze freely or a person with chickens in their backyard would not want to house their chickens indoors. Therefore, it is necessary to provide as many deterrents to natural predators of chickens as possible in outdoor facilities such as a chicken run.

A secure chicken coop where chickens are kept at night is the best way to protect chickens from predators. In addition to a coop with protection, the poultry run needs to be made as secure as possible. Predators will tunnel under the fencing in the run, jump over four foot fences and fly in and grab prey from the sky.

Fencing the chicken run

The fence around the poultry run is the most important deterrent for predators. As some predators such as bobcats can easily jump four foot fences so five or six feet high is better. There are a variety of materials that can be used for the fencing but it needs to be sturdy and the mesh needs to be fine so that cats and raccoons cannot reach in and grab a chicken. Minxes can get through very small mesh and so you will need a smaller mesh. Suggested materials include wire mesh, chicken wire, and welded wire mesh. Most agriculture departments recommend mesh that is 1-2" mesh or smaller. To protect chicken from flying predators such as hawks that attack in broad daylight and owls a good wire net cover is a good idea for covering the enclosure. The closure should also be made of fine mesh bird netting or welded wire material.

For the burrowing predator

Try burying hardware cloth that is galvanized around the perimeter of the enclosure. You can also use welded wire fencing around the edges in the same way to keep animals from tunneling into the chicken run.

Additional deterrents

Special lighting can be placed at strategic places that are motion sensor activated and are specifically for keeping predators at bay. There is even sound equipment to scare predators away. Try the use of objects that have motion such as pinwheels or flags or even scarecrows on or near the chicken run as they may be startling to animals. There are specially manufactured chemical products or pheromone substances that are made to repel certain types of predators that can be useful.

It will also help to keep shrubs or other vegetation absent from around the outside perimeter of the chicken run as animals don't like to be without cover when hunting. Keep the shrubs and vegetation within the enclosure and leave the outside fencing clear. It is fine to include shrubs and other toxic free plantings inside the enclosure for your chickens but keep the outside perimeter clear of plantings.

Your chicken coop will be more likely to protect your chickens if it is elevated. This will help prevent rodents, snakes or skunks from getting underneath the coop floor. It also helps in keeping these animals from raiding the chicken coop for eggs, hens or chicks. In addition, make sure that the floor of the chicken coop is kept in good repair to make it more difficult for a predator to get to the chickens.

To get the best results with the chicken coop once you are sure the building is secure is to make sure that all the chickens are closed up at night as they settle in to roost and to lay eggs.

If owls are a major predator in your area you might also want to get the chickens in the coop early before prime owl hunting time.

Chapter 7: How to Mate Chickens, Incubate Eggs and Hatch New Chicks

How do chickens mate?

Roosters like to mate with chickens that have big red combs and are in the prime of health. This is a biological instinct that keeps the best of the flock fertilized. Hens are not interested in new roosters but roosters are interested in new hens.

Hens like to mate with the dominant rooster and if by chance he is not there and the subdominant ones mate with the hens, the hen will eject the sperm and not get fertilized by the subdominant rooster. They cannot refuse the advances of the subdominant rooster but can reject the sperm. If the hen is approached by a rooster that is related to her she will automatically reject the sperm. The hen will also reject sperm if the rooster is not of good breed.

The male chicken will jump on the hen's back and holds her neck feathers with his beak. She will stoop a little so that she can bear his weight. He will tuck his tail below her body and shoot the sperm into the cloaca. The eggs will remain fertilized for 7 days. The rooster will decide how much sperm he will give the chicken. This will depend on the availability of hens to mate.

How many chickens to rooster ratio do you need if you want to breed chicks?

A good ratio is one rooster to 6 to 8 chickens.

Incubating and Hatching Eggs

Chicken eggs need 21 days to hatch. They can be hatched in an incubator or by a chicken sitting on the eggs. The advantages of having a broody chicken is that she will do everything herself and you will not have to do anything. However some eggs can get broken.

Without an incubator, a broody hen will hatch out eggs. They should not have more than 12 eggs under them or they will not be able to look after the eggs. A clutch of eggs is around 12. Japanese Silkies and Game bird hens are some of the best brooders. The game hens are especially good mothers.

The temperature of the incubator needs to be around 99 degrees. It must be around this temperature or the eggs will not hatch. The incubator must be checked and set to this temperature.

The eggs must be turned 2 to 3 times daily. The chicken will do this naturally when they sit on the eggs. If the eggs are being hatched by incubator they will be turned manually by you. After 18 days the eggs don't need to be turned.

Humidity should be at 60 to 65 percent during the first 18 days. This will be natural when a chicken sits on the eggs but must be properly maintained when using an incubator. You can raise the humidity by using a pan of water or some wet sponges. To decrease humidity you will need to have a smaller pan of water and fewer sponges.

Try not to open the door after the 18th day. As it is very critical not to disturb the eggs at this time or subject them to a change in temperature.

Which is better natural or artificial incubation?

Natural incubation with the hen sitting on the eggs is easiest and best for the chicks. The hen will take care of the eggs and protect the chicks. The only disadvantage is that a natural broody hen will not be able to hatch out as many eggs as an incubator.

However if you are prepared to keep the incubator at the right temperature and humidity, plus turn the eggs manually then an incubator is the next best thing. You will also have to look after the chicks when they hatch out. Additionally when the chicks are old enough you will need to introduce them to the flock. Chicks have special needs like keeping them warm and feeding them properly. They require quite a bit of care.

Chapter 8 : Steps on How to Introduce Chicks or New Chickens to the Old Flock

Introducing a new chicken to an established flock?

Several factors need to be considered when introducing new chickens to the flock. You must be very careful especially if you introduce chicks. Be aware that chickens are very territorial and have a specific pecking order that the flock will adhere to. The pecking order can be seen especially when the food comes into the run or coop. The dominant hen will take the food first and will be followed by the other hens in the order of dominance. Social animals and birds will all have this way of living. When new birds are introduced to the flock they will encounter fights and pecking from the older birds. Chicks can be pecked to death if not carefully introduced. You will need to wait until the chicks are full grown before introducing them to the flock. Never introduce a new rooster to the flock as there will be fights between him and the old rooster.

There is also a question of introducing disease to the old flock if the new birds are not properly watched before they join the flock. The easiest way to do this is to separate the chickens by creating a separate place for them. Clean the bottom of your shoes or boots before entering the old flock's territory. This will prevent any contamination. Keep the new flock separated from the old ones for several weeks. Be sure that they can see each other through the fence, so that they will get used to seeing each other.

To avoid fights and even death, introduce the new birds at night when the others are sleeping. There will be fewer fights when you do this. The new birds will take up the smell of the old ones at night. Also be sure to have enough room for the additions, so they can hide from the older birds if necessary. There will also be less fighting if the birds are not overcrowded.

Make sure the chicks are grown up and are the same size as the older birds before they are introduced to the old flock. Separating them, as mentioned above, will allow the chickens to see but not touch the new birds. You can put the pen inside the old run and allow the old birds to get used to seeing but not peck at the new birds. This will help to familiarize the two sets of birds. You can do this when the new flock have been carefully checked and quarantined for possible diseases.

Try to be sure there is enough food and drink, with plenty of room, so that the old birds will not guard all the food and water from the new birds and prevent them from eating and drinking. More than one container of food and water should be set out. You should feed and water the new flock before they join the old one.

You can create a diversion for the older birds by hanging corn cobs in accessible places. The older birds will be busy taking a peck at the corn instead of at the new birds. If any bird gets injured take them out as soon as you can and separate them until they are healed up. You can put anti pecking ointment on their wounds to prevent further pecking. Chickens will peck at blood and also pick on injured or weak chickens. This is an instinctive action to preserve the strength of the flock.

There is a pecking order that chickens will establish themselves. It is better not to interfere in this process. It is wise not to introduce a single chicken to the flock as this will stress out the newcomer and can even lead to her death.

Never introduce a new rooster to the flock if you have an established one. They will fight and possibly injure and kill each other. This is a territorial thing that all chickens, especially roosters will exhibit. The roosters will also fight for dominance and possession of the females. The strongest rooster will become the dominant one and will be given preference by the hens.

Chapter 9: Nutritious feeds and supplements for chicks and chickens

Natural food of chicks and chickens

Bear in mind that chickens are omnivores and not just vegetarian. This means that their natural diet will be grains, vegetables and meat protein. This translates to them having a variety of food.

Forage food: Chickens love to scratch about foraging for food. If you have free range birds they will do this naturally. Grass either cut or pulled is a favorite foraging food for chickens. The chicken droppings will mix up in the grass clippings and make good compost. Try to keep the clippings fresh.

Weeds are also a nice foraging food. You can have a run on wheels if you do not have too many chickens and put the chickens to work on any land you want weeded and tilled. They will scratch the ground and aerate it plus their droppings will act as good fertilizer. Additionally they will eat unwanted insects and clear the garden of pests and weeds. Chickens will eat up any plant and are quite indiscriminant about what they eat. Be sure there are no daffodils or morning glory, as these plants is poisonous for them. The chickens usually avoid these plants but you do not want to take any risk. You can also just throw weeds into the run and the chickens will eat them up happily.

Bugs and worms are also popular with chickens. Again they will eat a lot of garden pests if wheeled out to a particular area of your garden. Or better still just let them forage in the fall or before your spring plant.

All sorts of grains, especially corn and oats are good natural food for chickens. They will also eat table scraps. It is wise to cut these up and refrain from giving them chicken to eat.

What type of feed is the best to use for chicks?

In the natural way, the mother will lead the little chicks out and break all the food for them. This will include small seeds, grains and foraging food. However if you are just starting your flock, or do not have a mother hen to help your chicks, you must rely on the feed that you provide the chicks.

You can start them on chick starter feed from your local feed store or you can make your own. You can use these grains for feed: cracked shelled sunflower seeds, finely cracked wheat, finely cracked hulled (not pearl) barley, finely rolled oats, cornmeal, cracked rye, dandelion, millet, alfalfa seed etc. They also need greens like chopped lettuce, chard, kale, cabbage, wheatgrass and alfalfa sprouts.

How often do you need to feed newborn chicks?

Food and water should be available to the chicks at all times as they are birds and will spend most of their time sleeping, eating and drinking. Remember to get a proper drinking utensil and feeding container for them. This will ensure that food and drink will get spilt less and will always be available. Especially be careful that you give them a proper water container as they can get into the water and accidentally drown. You can get special feeders and water containers from your local feed store.

Chick food recipe

Chick mash is easier on the chick's digestive system and is made from 2 cups rolled oats, 4 cups cracked wheat, 1 cup finch seed and 1 cup cornmeal.

When the chicks are 2 days old you can add 1 cup of thistle mix and shelled, crushed sunflower seed.

If you wish to ferment the mash and make it a more digestible, mix it with enough water to cover and leave it for at least 8 hours.

Use ¼ cup of meat protein until the chicks are 3 weeks old. Use ½ cup after this. You can use cooked ground scraps.

When the chicks are 2 days old 1 cup of alfalfa sprouts can be added to the mix. You can add greens that are chopped up as the chicks get bigger. Dirt and oyster shells can be scattered on the floor so that the chicks will get used to foraging.

What type of foods is the best to use for chickens?

Natural food is best. However if you are feeding them commercial feed this is the régime, they will need a grower starter feed from 4 weeks to 6 months. Then they will have an egg layer feed. You can make your own feed for the chickens. You can also use grass clippings through the summer and weeds, which are good foraging food for the chickens. The chickens will forage through this and produce great fertilizer for spring planting. Be sure that it is fresh and do not use bagged grass clippings as they can have mold. You can grow your own greens for chickens.

These grains are good for chicken feed: corn, amaranth ("pig weed"), buckwheat, wheat, oats, cowpeas, rye and barley.

A good mix of grains, vegetables and foraging food will be good for growing feed and egg laying feeds. It is better for the chickens and the eggs you eat.

Extra protein should help them to get over the molting period more quickly and help them recover if they are sick. Cat food from a can that is ground up can help supply more protein. If they begin to peck at each other and eat their eggs, this can be a sign of lack of calcium. They can be given ground up oyster shells to give them more calcium. Calcium supplements can be given. Stones and small pieces of gravel known as grits must always be provided when chickens are fed. This is because they do not have teeth and everything passes through the gizzard, which helps to grind the food. Ground oyster shells are good for this purpose. If the birds have an outside run where they can forage they will instinctively pick up small stones and gravel for their gizzards.

How many times a day should you feed your chickens?

Chickens are birds and as such will pick up small morsels of food all day. The best way to keep them well-fed is to set them out in the run to forage and keep the feeder available as well. Put it in the shade on hot sunny days. A little ice in their water for really hot days is nice.

Is dry food enough for your chickens?

Dry food made from the grains mentioned above is good for your chickens but they also need foraging foods to remain in the peak of health. Vegetables like kale and lettuce are also good for them as they give the birds valuable minerals and vitamins. They will also need grit like ground up oyster shells.

Will putting methylene blue in their water be good for them?

Methylene blue is used mainly in fish tanks to stop fungus in the water and rotting of unfertilized eggs. It is not necessary to put this substance in the water unless the chickens are getting fungal infections. If they are suffering from any disease like thrush it is a good idea to use methylene blue in their water. Usually regular tap water is alright for chickens to drink.

How do you keep up the water supply?

The best way to keep the chickens with a good water supply is to have one or two containers of water in the run or coop. You can get a special water feeder for your chicks and also for chickens. It is best to change the water every day and clean the water utensil at least every week to prevent mold. If winters are very cold you may need a small heater that fits below the water container. In extreme summers some ice in the water container for the chickens is a nice thing to do. Also place the water in the shade if possible.

What feeds do you recommend to keep eggs "organic" and all natural?

The all natural recipe mentioned below is a good standard feed for chickens. They should also be allowed to forage if possible, as this is their natural food. If they cannot forage due to weather and other factors then as well as their grain diet they should be given leafy vegetables like kale and lettuce.

Do hens need a special type of food to lay eggs?

Commercially fed hens will have a feed called egg mash. Naturally fed hens can have the recipe below plus foraging food.

How do you make chicken feeds?

Here is a good nutritious natural feed for your chickens. It is a good supplement for foraging foods especially in winter when foraging can become less rewarding for the chickens.

A recipe for chicken food

3 parts soft white wheat
2 parts whole corn
3 parts hard red winter wheat
½ part Diatomaceous Earth edible kind that the chickens can use for grit
2 part sunflower seeds
1 part hulled barley
1 part oat groats
1 part wheat bran
1 part split peas
½ part peanuts
1 part quinoa
1 part sesame seeds
1 part lentils
1/2 part kelp

Mix all the ingredients by hand. Make sure it is fresh and stored in an airtight container.

Chapter 10: Tips to Keep Your Chicks and Chickens Healthy

Keeping Your Chickens Healthy

Your first tactic is to keep the coop clean. You will need to do a deep clean every week to make sure that the chickens are healthy and happy. Be sure to take all the nesting boxes out of the coop and give them a detailed cleaning. Remove all the old bedding and replace it with new clean bedding. Scrub the roosts down and remember to clean the perches with a 50/50 solution of vinegar and water. Spray a citrus spray to make the coop smell sweet and kill bacteria. A recipe is given on the previous chapter. Be sure to scrub the walls and floor with the vinegar solution to cut down bacteria and parasites and be sure to check for pests when removing the old bedding.

Food and water should be changed daily. It is important to keep these fresh so that there is no infection. You should clean all water and food utensils once a week. Scrub down the containers with the 50/50 vinegar solution. The vinegar will not harm the chickens as it is a natural product. This will prevent many common diseases of chickens and keep the flock healthy and happy.

Make sure there is good ventilation inside the coop. This is very important as chickens are dusty animals and are very susceptible to respiratory diseases. It is also good to keep them comfortable with a good air flow. This will cut down bacteria and virus infections as the germs will not breed so well if there is a good flow of air.

Always allow enough space for your chickens. Overcrowding can lead to stress and even cannibalism. Chickens are territorial birds and will need at least 8 feet of space per medium sized bird. They will also remain healthier if they have enough space.

Separate any chickens that fall sick. Firstly, they can spread infection to the other healthy members of the flock. Secondly, the other chicken will pick upon a sick chicken and may even kill it. This is because they will do this instinctively to keep the flock healthy and strong.

Is it better to let them free range or be in a run that you can move?

If you have a garden, it is good to have a movable run. This is also known as a tractor run. You can take it out to different parts of the garden that need tilling and clearing. The chickens will have fun and get exercise and you will have a well-prepared area of your garden. The chickens will take care of the pests and all plants that are not protected from them. A small flock of just six birds will do a great job of clearing and tiling land in just a few days. They will also provide fertilizer to the garden area. Be sure that the run is big enough for your flock and that they cannot escape into other parts of the garden.

If you do not have a need for chickens to take care of your garden then a permanent run is best. You can throw weeds, fresh grass clippings and vegetables in the run for foraging food to supplement their feed.

Do chickens need to be out of their coops too?

Yes, chickens do need to be out of their coop. The best way to manage this is to build a   run for them to take exercise and forage for food. They will have less stress and there   will be less fighting in the coop if they are managed this way.

A tractor coop is good if you want land prepared for a garden. You need to be sure that   it is big enough for the chickens to take exercise and enjoy foraging for little tidbits.

The nesting boxes and roosts can be in the coop but the chickens need a break from the   chicken house. They will be happier and healthier if they have a run. Chickens who spend their entire lives in the coop will exhibit signs of stress.

Aside from food and water, what are the other things that chicks and chickens need?

They need a clean coop and a run if possible. Keeping the coop clean is essential for good hygiene and healthy birds. A run will let the chicken take exercise and forage. It will also reduce stress for the chicken.

They also need space, about 4 square feet per chicken. Chickens are birds and therefore are territorial. For this reason they need space. This will also reduce stress for the chicken.

Nesting boxes are good and roosts are necessary. Again because chickens are birds they will like to roost above ground. This will prevent predators and pests from attacking the chickens. They will also be more comfortable. Nesting boxes are good for egg layers so that they will not lay their eggs in different places where you cannot find them. To encourage the use of nesting boxes, place a dummy egg in there at first. Always leave one egg in the nesting box so that the chicken feels that it is a safe place to lay eggs. Chickens do not count but do notice if an egg is in the nest or not.

Clean dry bedding: This is very important for the comfort and health of the chicken. For deep manure method for heating the coop in winter just keep adding bedding. You will also get cleaner eggs, if you keep bedding and nesting boxes clean.

The coop should be well-protected against predators and pests that can bother the chickens.

Reducing the Stress Levels of Your Chickens

Chickens can face stress like any other animal. This can be translated into fighting and picking on each other. It can also result in egg breaking and eating. There are a number of ways that chickens can get stressed out.

Staying inside the coop: Chickens will get stressed if they are kept inside continuously. They like to run around and forage for food and grit for their gizzards. It is best to build them a run and let them out during the day. You should only keep them in the coop at night time.

Keep them warm and dry: If their living quarters are comfortable and dry the chickens will be happier and less stressed. Be sure your coop is well-ventilated so that ammonia does not build up in the coop.

Cut down noise: Brooding hens need peace and quiet. Try to decrease noise around the hen house where the brooding hen is.

Herbs: Herbs mixed with the bedding can have a soothing effect on the chicken.

Chapter 11: Most Common Chicken Diseases and Problems

Backyard chickens are usually quite healthy. You should call the vet and get them vaccinated when they are chicks so that they remain healthy. The key to keeping your chickens in good health is keeping the coop clean and making sure that you change the water and food daily. If you do this and let your chickens out in a well protected run you should not have any problems but diseases can afflict your flock and you need to be prepared.

Most common diseases for chicks

- **Coccidiosis**

This is caused by protozoa that are passed from one chick to another in the stool of the chick. This disease can be treated by giving the chicks medicated feed. The feeder and water container should be properly cleaned and disinfected and clean water and food should be provided daily.

- **Pullorium**
  Chicks are usually very active and continuously cheep, except when they are sleeping. If you notice a chick that is not as active as the rest then it is good to keep an eye on it. The chick will also have a white diarrhea with paste that sticks to their rear ends. They can also experience breathing difficulties or die without displaying any symptoms. It is important to buy chicks from Pullorium-negative flocks.

- **Omphalitis (Mushy Chick)**

  This usually affects newly hatched chicks. The chicks appear enlarged, with a bluish tinge and inflammation of the navel area. The chicks are drowsy and weak and they smell unpleasant. They contract this illness from dirty surfaces or from other infected birds. The chick can have a navel infection resulting from a weak immune system. Treatment can be done by properly cleaning their housing and giving antibiotics. Often the chicks will die when they have this illness. Healthy chicks should be separated from the sick ones. There is no vaccine for this. The staph and strep germs that cause this problem can also make humans sick.

Common Diseases for Adult Chickens

- **Fowl pox**

This can be seen as white spots on the skin and sores with scabs on their combs. They can also have white ulcers in the mouth and in their trachea. Egg laying will cease. It is caused by a virus.

Treatment: keep their living quarters warm and dry and give them soft food. With good care the birds can recover.

- **Botulism**

The chicken will experience tremors and will become paralyzed. Their lungs will also stop working and they will be dead in a few hours. Feathers can be pulled out easily. This disease can be contracted by drinking or eating botulism contaminated food and water. You can treat it with a teaspoon of Epsom salts in 1 ounce of warm water and feed it to the bird several times in the day. Remove the source of contamination and change the chickens' water and food every day. No vaccine is available for this infection.

- **Fowl Cholera**

Chickens over 4 months can be infected by this disease. They will exhibit greenish yellow diarrhea and swollen joints. The head and wattles will become darkened and they will have difficulty in breathing. They will often die quickly. All the chickens that are infected should be destroyed as even if a bird recovers it will become a carrier. This is a very contagious disease. It can be contracted by rats, raccoons, opossums and wild birds. Contaminated soil, clothing, shoes or equipment can also carry the bacteria that cause this disease. Water and food can also carry the disease if they become contaminated. There is no treatment for this and only the State Department of Agriculture can administer vaccinations.

- **Infectious Bronchitis**

  This can be seen when a chicken is sneezing, wheezing and has watery discharge from eyes and nose. The hens will stop laying. This is an extremely contagious disease and can be spread by contaminated surfaces, air and from bird to bird. If chicks contract this disease, they will have 50% mortality if they are less than 6 weeks. Vaccine should be administered to the hens before they are 15 weeks old.

- **Infectious Coryza**

  Chickens will exhibit swollen wattles, combs and swollen heads. Their nose and eyes have a sticky discharge and eyes have so much swelling that they are shut. The chickens will also have areas of moisture under their wings. This disease is contracted from birds that are carriers, drinking water and contaminated surfaces. This is another disease where birds with the disease must be destroyed as they will carry the disease if they recover. There is no vaccine for this infection.

- **Marek's Disease**

  This disease will affect chicks and birds under 20 weeks. The chickens will develop tumors internally and externally. They will also experience paralysis. The iris of the eyes will become grey and not react to light. This is a very contagious disease and the birds will contract it by inhaling feather dust and skin cells from birds with this disease. There is no treatment for this and the death rate is high. Any surviving birds will be carriers of the disease. The chicks are usually vaccinated against this illness at 1 day old.

- **Moniliasis (Thrush)**

The chicken will show signs of a white cheesy substance around the crop. Their laying will be down and their feathers will be droopy and ruffled. They will have an increase in appetite. This is a fungal disease that can be contracted by the chickens eating moldy food and bad water. If surfaces have been contaminated by birds with this problem it can be transferred to other birds. It can occur after birds have received antibiotics for an unrelated problem. Water containers should be disinfected and fresh food should be provided. There is no vaccine for this problem.

- **Mycoplasmosis/CRD/Air Sac Disease**:

  When it is mild, the chicken will exhibit weakness and their laying will be down. However in its acute form the chicken's joints will swell and become infected. They will also have coughing, sneezing and breathing problems which can result in death. It can be contracted from wild birds and can be transmitted through the egg to the chick if the mother hen has the disease. It is important to see the vet if your chicken displays these symptoms and they may recommend a course of antibiotics. There is a vaccine for this illness.

- **Newcastle Disease**

  The chicken will display symptoms of wheezing and will have difficulty in breathing. Laying will stop. They will have cloudy eyes and have twisted necks and heads. Their legs are paralyzed and also their wings. It is very contagious and can be contracted from wild birds as well as infected chickens, shoes, clothes and any surfaces that have been in contact with the disease. Birds less than 6 months often die but older ones may recover. The recovered chickens are not carriers. There is a vaccine for this disease.

- **Pullorum**

Older birds will have poor laying capacity and have signs of sneezing and coughing. This disease is contracted through carrier birds, clothing, shoes and contaminated surfaces. The only treatment is to destroy the birds that are infected as even those who recover become carriers. There is no vaccine to prevent this disease.

How do external parasites affect chicks and chickens?

The external parasites that can affect you chicks and chickens can make them very uncomfortable and if not checked can even lead to death. The worst offenders are lice and mites. Chickens can also be exposed to fleas and ticks. These parasites are more prevalent in the warm season and can multiply quickly.

- **Lice**
  These parasites are found on the feathers and skin of a chicken. They feast on feather parts, blood and dry skin scales. They do not live on humans but can be very irritating to the chicken. There are different types of lice that are named because of where they are found on the body. Shaft and neck louse are some of the most common.

It is important to catch these parasites early. They are most prevalent in warmer months. You can check for these parasites once a week in summer and about once a month in the cooler months. You should spread the feathers of the chicken so that you can see the skin and feather shafts of the neck, vent and wings of the bird. You should also be able to see the skin and base of the feathers of the chicken. Eggs will appear as white clusters and the adult lice will be 3 mm in length and brown in color. If one of the chickens has lice then the rest will probably be infected. The best treatment is dusting with lice powder. It will kill all the adults and when you dust 7 days later, it will kill all the baby lice that have hatched out.

- **Mites**
  There are 3 common types of mites that can affect your chickens, the Scaly Leg Mite, Northern Fowl Mite and Red Mites. They can also affect humans.

Red Mites

Red mites are very small and nocturnal so they are difficult to see. They are pale grey and turn bright red after eating. The mites can be found in the cracks and crevices of the walls and roosts. They are potentially dangerous to the chickens and should not be allowed to fester. Chickens may even be disinclined to roost at night. You should dust the birds, but the whole chicken coop should be cleaned in detail and dusted with Red Mite powder.

Northern Fowl Mites

They can attack the chickens in the day or night and are also potentially dangerous for the chickens. They can result in anemia and even death of the birds. The Northern Fowl Mites are more prevalent in winter than in warmer months. They are brown or black in color. Treatment is done by dusting the birds with mite powder.

Scaly Leg Mites

These mites burrow under the chickens scales on their legs and feet. The scales of the chicken' feet and legs become swollen and distorted. White crusts can develop on the scales and the scales themselves can even fall off. The chicken will feel a lot of discomfort. These mites can spread rapidly so you will need to clean the coop thoroughly. You can treat the chickens in several ways. One is to cover their legs with Vaseline or benzyl benzoate. You can dip the chicken's legs in surgical spirit twice per week.

- **Poultry Ticks**
  These ticks are more prevalent in wooden chicken coops. The eggs of the ticks can be dormant for years. They hide in cracks and crevices during the day and feed on the chickens at night. They will weaken the affected chicken and can kill birds if they are allowed to fester. The chickens will eat them if they find the ticks.

- **Fleas**:

  These parasites can be found in the run or chicken coop. They will cause restlessness and discomfort to the chicken. It is not good for broody hens to have fleas as they can make the hen uncomfortable and when she moves around she may break the eggs. Treatment can be done with a good flea dusting powder and attention to cleaning the coop well.

  It is very difficult to eradicate these external parasites. It is best to check the birds regularly and keep the coop and all accessories like roosts and nesting boxes clean.

What do you do if the egg got cracked or get stuck inside the bird?

Egg binding can be a serious problem for the chicken. It is when an egg gets stuck in the ovarian tract. This will prevent the chicken from laying and needs to be addressed or the chicken may die. You can gently massage the hen to coax the egg out. If this fails then it is best to call the vet. The vet will break the egg and bring it out in pieces. When this is done, the ovary tract must be cleaned well to prevent any injuries from broken pieces of shell or infections due to parts of the egg getting contaminated.

There are a few causes of egg binding. One of the main ones is lack of calcium and Vitamin D. The hens should be fed a calcium rich diet and you can supplement their feed with calcium supplements like ground oyster shells. You can also use a calcium mineral block.

In winter time, in areas where the weather is extremely cold and the chickens have less sunlight, they can suffer from lack of vitamin D. You can use full spectrum lighting to provide valuable UVA and UVB rays. There are also food supplements that contain vitamin D.

Before using supplements always consult your vet as too much vitamin D can cause kidney damage.

Lack of protein can also attribute to egg binding problems. This can happen if the birds are fed on a seed only diet. Cooked beans and rice are good for your birds and provide extra protein. Cooked meats and sea food can also be used. Do not use soy protein supplements as they have too many probiotics. It is wise not to use dairy products, or yogurt.

Proper nutrition and clean food and water should take care of this problem. If it is a persistent problem then you should consult your vet.

What do you do if the hens lay soft-shelled, thin-layered shell or misshapen eggs?

Misshapen eggs are often seen when young chickens start laying. They will generally improve in shape and size when the hen has been laying eggs for awhile. However there are some other underlying causes that you should be aware of.

A sudden drop in egg production with established egg laying hens can be an indication of disease. The eggs may be misshapen when this occurs. You need to check the hen carefully for any signs of disease and treat them if necessary.

Heat and high or low humidity levels can also cause this problem. The coop should be well-ventilated to avoid a build up of humidity. The doors of the coop should be opened during the day time and face the run. This means that there will be less humidity built up.

Parasites and toxins like mold can also affect the eggs. The water for the chickens should be changed daily as should the food. The coop should be cleaned well to avoid build up of molds and parasites. Check the chickens on a daily basis to be sure that they are healthy.

Molting and stress can also cause egg problems. Extra protein can be added to the diet when the chickens are in molt.

This can happen also due to lack of calcium. The remedy for this is to give them ground up oyster shells, which you can sprinkle on the food. A calcium block can also be used and vegetables that provide calcium can be given to the chickens. The chickens can also suffer from lack of vitamin B12, E and D. They can also have deficiencies of calcium, selenium and phosphorus, which can affect the shells of laying hens. These deficiencies can result in soft shells, thin shells or absence o a shell.

What do you do if your chickens eat their own eggs?

Again this is a lack of calcium. Use the calcium supplements mentioned above. If the chickens get into a habit of eating eggs you should keep the chicken away from the flock. Keep the nesting box dark so that the chicken does not see the egg and remove the egg as soon as possible. Once they get out of the habit they can return to the flock.

Chapter 12: Ways to Care for a Sick Chicken

Signs and Symptoms of a Sick Chicken

The first thing you may notice is a decline or even complete stopping of egg production. When the chicken is not in molt, or at a rest time in their egg cycle, you should be aware that something might be wrong. Chickens will display signs of not eating or drinking. They will also exhibit symptoms of the actual disease. There are certain other obvious signs.

If a chicken is sitting quietly with her wings drooping and she is not broody. You will know the difference because a broody hen will fluff up her feathers and get angry when you approach. A sick bird will not react in this way. She will be sitting away from the flock and will remain depressed and quiet when you approach.

She has a heavy infestation of lice. Normally a chicken will get rid of many lice and will not get heavily infested. However if they are sick lice can accumulate quickly.

Coughing and wheezing can also be a symptom of the chicken not being well. In fact this is a symptom of a number of fatal diseases so you need to be careful if you see this.

Diarrhea or no stool is an indication that something is not right.

Limping or moving around in an uncomfortable way can indicate the chicken has swollen painful joints. This is another indication of serious disease and should be seen to as soon as possible.

Discharge or bleeding from the vent is another symptom of something serious.

Do you need to isolate the sick chickens from the healthy ones?

There are two reasons for separating sick chickens from the healthy ones. Firstly, you do not want the other birds to get any problems. Many of the diseases a chicken can get are quite contagious and can spread quickly to the rest of the flock. Secondly, chickens will also pick on a sick chicken and can peck it to death. This is an instinctive method that chickens and birds have to keep the flock strong.

Where do you buy medicines for your sick chickens?

You can purchase medicine for sick chickens at your local feed store. The vet can also supply medicines for your flock, if needed. Antibiotics and other medicines can also be purchased online.

Do chickens get sick easily?

Backyard chickens are usually quite healthy. You should call the vet and get them vaccinated so that they remain well. There are some common ailments that do afflict chickens but usually they remain in good health.

Chapter 13: Effective steps to increase egg production

Ways to increase or initiate egg production and quality of eggs

Chickens will start to lay at around 6 months of age. To keep egg laying at maximum production you can use these techniques:

To encourage laying and to keep a chicken using a nesting box, you can keep one egg in the box or use a glass egg. The chicken will then get used to laying in that place and will not move around. If they do not see an egg in the nesting box, they will feel that the place is not safe and will lay in a different place.

Let the chickens out after 10 a.m. as they will have finished their laying by this time and you will not have to search for the eggs outside.

Feed the chickens well with nutritious organic food. Let them out for a run to forage as this will reduce stress and help to keep egg laying production to an optimum level.
If you are feeding with commercial food use an egg laying feed.

Happy, healthy chickens will lay better. It is good to keep a good supply of fresh food and water and keep their coop clean.

Be sure you choose the right egg laying breeds for your area. There are certain breeds like Rhode Island Reds and Leghorns that will lay well.

Be sure to put a light in the coop in winter to stimulate egg laying.

What kind of light makes chickens lay more eggs?

Any light will stimulate them to lay in winter. In order to be sure that the chickens will continue to lay, you will need to keep lights in the chicken coop for around 12 to 14 hours per day. As the days start shortening start using the lights, a timer is good so that you do not have to spend time turning the light on and off.

Do chickens prefer to lay eggs in the dark?

Chickens like private places to lay their eggs as they want them to be safe from predators. Some chickens will seek out private dark places others do not care and will even lay in the open if allowed. It is good to have one nesting box per hen as they like to lay eggs in the same place if possible. This gives them a little privacy. Make a perch near the box so that they can hop in easily.

How warm do chickens need to be in order for them to lay eggs?

Ideally in winter, if weather is very severe, you can use a heat lamp and keep the coop at around 50 degrees. Chickens naturally fluff out their feathers and keep themselves warm, without help from you. They also huddle together if it gets chilly. The deep litter method will also keep the coop warm and comfortable. If it gets too hot the chicken may not lay eggs until the weather cools down.

Does playing music affect the rate at which chickens lay their eggs?

There is quite a bit of controversy about music being played in the coop and whether it really helps with egg production. Some people say that certain music will keep the chickens calm and help with egg laying production. Others feel that it makes no difference.

Factors that affect the hens when they lay eggs

Light is a big factor. Chickens have an inborn instinct to lay fewer eggs as the days get shorter. Placing a timer light will help to keep egg production up. Their health is another factor. The breed of the hen is also important as some breeds have been specially bred for egg production. Leghorns, Rhode Island Reds and Austalorps are good egg laying breeds.

Good nutrition will also help the hens to lay better. Be sure to feed them extra protein when they are laying eggs. Commercial egg laying mash can be used or a mixture of grains and seeds with a supplement of green leafy vegetables. Remember to supplement their diet with calcium supplements to ensure that their eggs do not have thin or no shell.

Keeping your hens happy and healthy will ensure better egg laying. Chickens that are healthy and happy will lay more eggs than those that are not in the peak of health. You should check the flock regularly to make sure that they do not have any ailments or parasites, as both these factors can lower egg production.

Clean food and water will also be a factor. Change the water and food daily.

Try to maintain a clean well -ventilated coop. Keeping the coop clean and ensuring that they have clean water and food will also help to kelp the chickens healthy and laying well.

Chapter 14: Checklist of Chores You Need to Do Daily to Manage Healthy and Happy Chickens

Daily and over-all responsibilities of the chicken coop owner

A light clean up should be performed daily. You can place shelves under roosts to collect droppings. These can be removed and cleaned everyday.

After 10 a.m. eggs can be collected. You may have to collect eggs more often if the weather is warmer so that they do not get spoiled.

Food and water should be replaced on a daily basis. This will cut down diseases.

Check the flock to make sure they are all active and healthy. You should also check them for external parasites every week.

You should open the coop door to the run every morning and close it securely every evening. This will aerate the coop and help to ventilate it. Remember to check the coop on a regular basis to be sure that it is predator proof.

If your winters are very cold you should take precautions to heat the coop with a heat lamp, or use another method of heating the coop. You can use a timer or manually take care of the lighting on a daily basis.

As winter days get short, you should keep a light in the coop so that the chickens will have at least 14 hours of light. This will ensure that egg laying will not be drastically reduced.